A Guide To Prostate Cancer

"From A Survivor, What To Expect In 2020"

R.J. Mauro

Printed in the United States of America

First Printing, 2020

ISBN # 9798681914389

RJ Mauro

California, United States

prostatecancer1965@gmail.com

Mission and Disclosure

My mission is to simply inform as many people as possible about prostate cancer . My hope is that whoever reads my story will share it with as many people as possible as well.

Please keep in mind that I am NOT a doctor nor am I offering you any advice whatsoever about treatment options for your prostate cancer. I am simply sharing my experience with my own prostate cancer in hopes to make your experience a little easier.

All of your treatment options will be made by your urologist and health care team based on your diagnosis and your level of prostate cancer, and a whole host of other factors. The treatments that you choose to go with will be a decision made by you and your loved ones.

I hope you find this extremely useful .

Table of Contents

About Me

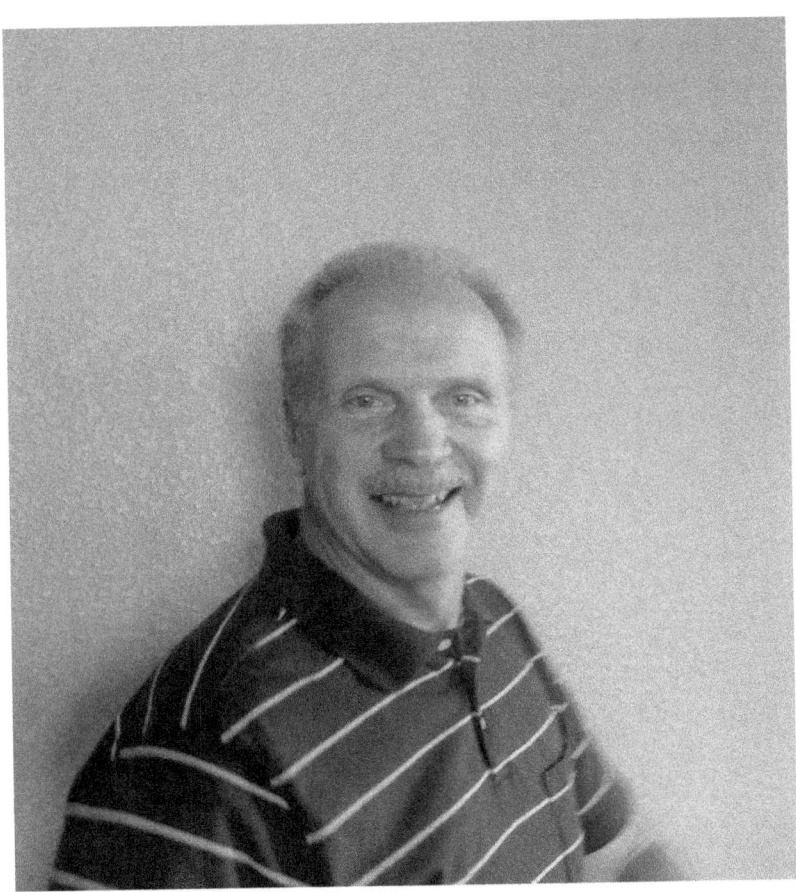

Just so you get an idea about who I am . My name is Ray and I'm a 54 year old truck driver from California.

I am married to a great woman who takes great care of me and our family.
We were married in 2005 and have been together since 2002.
Together we have 6 children, all grown, and 7 grandchildren and

twins on the way at the time I wrote this. The twins are due at the end of Nov 2020 or beginning of Dec 2020.

I wanted to provide you with a quick guide to help you to know exactly what might be ahead for you in the coming days and weeks with your own prostate cancer diagnosis.

Use this guide for yourself or pass it on to someone you know who might be going through this as well. Just pass it on to anyone you know.

Prostate Cancer Stats

Every year in the United States around 200,000 men are diagnosed with prostate cancer. You can find more statistics here
Prostate Cancer Stats In The USA

Worldwide prostate cancer tops 1 million men diagnosed per year . You can find worldwide statistics on prostate cancer here .
Worldwide Prostate Cancer Stats

The fact of the matter with prostate cancer in men is , it is the 2nd leading cause of death in men worldwide next to skin cancer .
And it is the 5th leading cause of death overall for men and women .

Keep in mind that almost 30,000 men die in the United States alone each year from prostate cancer. Early detection and good prostate health is key and easy .
Worldwide deaths from prostate cancer each year tops 300,000.

You can help lower these statistics for men by sharing information like this with your friends and family . Early detection can save lives .
Getting younger men on board with prostate health is also a key factor in reducing prostate cancer diagnosis and death .

There is more information on starting on prostate health early at the link below.

Get Started Here With Early Prostate Health!

Prostate Cancer Treatments

After consulting with your primary doctor and urologist regarding your symptoms and prostate exam findings , you will be presented with choices for treatment by your care team .
Based on what they find your choices will most likely be radiation or surgery , or a combination of both.
I will talk about my own treatment options later.

Radiation in 2020 is highly effective and very accurate, however , if radiation is

done and surgery is still needed , radiation makes surgery a bit more difficult due to scar tissue is what I am told. Check it out for yourself, as always your own research is best.

My Early Symptoms

My symptoms began quite a while before I had my first PSA TEST.
As a truck driver I am required to have a physical every 2 years.
Each time I took this physical it included a urine test and mine always
had "trace blood"
In my urine.
The doctor always said " get it checked out" and I did nothing.

Then about a year before surgery my symptoms changed . My urine flow
began slowing and even occasionally stopping mid stream . I also had
frequent urges to go pee more often. And a few months before that
something else started around the same time , I'll get into that speculation
in a later post .

So , trace blood in my urine for several years.
And about a year before surgery my urges to go pee more frequently and
a weak stream , occasionally stopping mid stream.
Those were my enlarged prostate or prostate symptoms.

My Family History

If you don't know yet , I'm 54 years old and just went through prostate cancer surgery August 19 , 2020.
54 years old is pretty young for prostate cancer. The vast majority of men diagnosed are over 60 years old.
Genetics had much to do with my diagnosis.

My father had prostate cancer at around 60 years old . I was not aware at the time that I should be tested for it, so I didn't .
If one of your male family members has had prostate cancer, your dad or grandfather you need to be tested .
Even your mom's dad and his dad . Get tested.

If you do in fact have prostate cancer the facility that you get treated at may be able to do some genetic testing for you and look for the gene .
Then you can pass on this info to your son's and their sons .

So my situation was definitely genetic and nothing else.
If you do have a family member history of prostate cancer you should be tested as soon as possible.

Remember ... 30,000 men die from prostate cancer each year in the United States. Early detection is way better than waiting.
My own situation is definitely a testament to that.

How I Found Out That I Have Prostate Cancer

I guess if I hadn't found out that I have prostate cancer when I did , I probably would have died from it given the severity of my cancer .

In late January 2020 my wife and I started shopping for life insurance. We zeroed in on a company for $400,000 in coverage on my life . We went through the process and the last step was a phlebotomist came out to our home and drew blood for standard tests . PSA TEST being one of them .

And Boom ! There it was , a PSA score over the high end of the good range . 4 being the high end of good . Mine was 4.75 . And with that we were turned down for the insurance policy.

From that life insurance PSA TEST I then scheduled a meeting with my doctor . Covid-19 had hit now and I had a video visit with my doctor . And sent him all of the blood test results from the insurance company.

My primary doctor referred me to a urologist for a prostate exam and another PSA TEST to confirm. The physical prostate exam was described as my prostate felt "dense" ... Not soft . From there my urologist and I set up a full prostate cancer biopsy to get a dozen tissue samples from the prostate.

And that's how I found out that I have prostate cancer.

Prostate Exam and Early Detection

As I mentioned in another post , early detection and good prostate health methods can be key to saving your life .

There is a whole host of prostate health information online and from your doctor.

One that I have recommended to my friends and family , namely my grown sons is this one . Good Prostate Health Here

It's all natural and promotes complete prostate health .

Early detection comes in 3 forms .

#1 a PSA blood test ordered by your primary care doctor. The PSA TEST is the standard blood test to detect possible prostate cancer. A PSA score above 4 is a possible sign of prostate cancer. However , not all scores above 4 are in fact prostate cancer.

#2 a prostate exam by your urologist. With 2 fingers and lasting only a few seconds or a minute at most ,your urologist can feel if your prostate is large , dense , or has a lump that doesn't belong there. A simple prostate exam can back up the PSA TEST score .

#3 Finally the prostate biopsy is the final early detection tool used by your urologist to determine if you have prostate cancer or not.

Prostate Biopsy is basically a scope inserted into the rectum with a camera and a small needle used to take around 12 small tissue samples from the prostate.

The needle penetrates through the wall of the colon into the prostate.

Super small holes . And a core sample is ejected into a tray . The samples are tested for cancer .

I'll go into my biopsy experience next

My Prostate Biopsy

The prostate biopsy for me was probably the most uncomfortable out of everything else I have been through since my first PSA test.
The biopsy comes after the regular prostate exam , if your doctor finds something they don't like during the exam .

So you schedule the biopsy and the night before or the morning of your biopsy you take prescription antibiotics . Mine were pretty powerful . In fact I got up to go pee in the middle of the night and I passed out in my bathroom. First time I ever passed out in my life. I let my doctor know and now that drug is listed as "I am allergic to it".

The antibiotics are to stop infection of course. But more specifically , during a prostate biopsy the needle goes through the wall of the colon into the prostate. Tiny needle and super fast . But it does punch a small hole into the wall of the colon . So when you poop, feces can get into the small holes and cause infection. That did not happen to me and is usually rare.

During the biopsy a nurse prepares you for the procedure. You undress and put on a gown . You lay down on your side and raise your knees towards your chest and try to relax.

The nurse puts a numbing gel in and around your rectum and then the doctor comes in.
Your doctor will explain what they will be doing.
The device will go into your rectum and the doctor will be able to see your prostate on screen .

Then they will start taking samples , maybe 12 core samples . 6 on each side of the prostate.

You'll feel a poke of the needle and hear a click of the trigger releasing the core sample into a tray.
The worst part is the doctor moving the instrument around to access the different areas of your prostate to get a sample. To me it felt like he was moving the joystick of a fighter jet in a dog fight! It was a pretty rough procedure to me.

The procedure is definitely uncomfortable, I was tensed up the entire time.
But the good news is it only lasted about 8 minutes .

My Final Prostate Cancer Diagnosis

Well this was my follow up visit with my urologist after the biopsy. It was a pretty rough day. Although I kinda knew what he was going to say to me, I had no idea to what extent my prostate cancer was at, and that was the hard part for me, and my wife.

I got there about 10 minutes early as usual and pretty much was called in without any waiting.
I got weighed and did a urine sample as usual, went into an exam room and got my blood pressure done and waited just a few minutes for my urologist.

My doctor came in and sat down and asked how I was , I said I was doing good. He then said … " I got the pathology report back on all the samples, pretty much every sample is cancer, not only that , but every one has a 7 , 8 , or 9 Gleason score. " The higher the score is not good.

You can read about Gleason Scores Here

I was kinda floored about what he was saying. He also said " this is not typical" "it's not good" "i'm concerned"
I think I was in some kind of fog , trying to grasp that he was saying I have cancer and it's not good. In fact he was saying the level of prostate cancer that I have is pretty bad.

I started to make jokes, my way of dealing with it.

My wife was out in the car and I knew she wasn't going to take it jokingly . This was pretty bad news for us. In an instant you are faced with your mortality which just 5 minutes earlier you really hadn't considered. Crazy stuff !

So the doctor ordered a pelvic MRI and a complete Bone Scan to see if the cancer had spread since my entire prostate was cancer. He also referred me to a surgical urologist. After that I left the office and headed out to the car.

I got to the car and got in . I knew my wife and family had been praying for it not to be cancer so this was gonna hurt. I also had to add that it was pretty bad cancer.
So I told her and we both started to cry and just hugged each other for a few minutes.
Keep in mind that this level of prostate cancer is usually for men in their 60s , not 54 .
It was pretty devastating information to take in.

But we did take it in and of course had no choice but to move forward. And everything from that moment on has moved pretty fast.

Here is a timeline since my video visit with my primary care doctor in 2020

May 27th video visit with primary care dr to discuss high PSA from insurance blood test.
July 6th office visit with urologist , prostate exam
July 9th prostate biopsy
July 20th follow up , review pathology , prostate cancer
August 3rd follow up after MRI and Bone Scan , No evidence of cancer spread
August 6th First meeting with surgeon
August 10th Primary care dr for pre op ekg , cardiac clearance
August 17th Covid-19 test 2 days before surgery

August 19th prostatectomy surgery.

In between the visits were the additional blood tests and imaging scheduled . It's been rough the past 3 months.

As I write this I'm in recovery from surgery just 9 days . Today is August 28, 2020 5:11pm pacific time .

Treatment Options For Me

The level of cancer in my prostate is pretty bad. I pretty much have only one option , and that is a prostatectomy. Removing my entire prostate. And that is what I chose to do without question.
I did have the option of doing radiation , but as I said earlier , radiation makes surgery a bit more challenging if you need surgery after radiation.

In my case , my care team basically told me my level of cancer needed removal. As I spoke with my urologist about my options we went over my questions about surgery.
I wasn't sure about what type of surgery I would be getting . I had looked up prostate surgery on google and youtube and I was seeing the robotic method with the DaVinci equipment . And the regular surgery called perineal prostatectomy.

I mentioned that to my urologist and he said " we don't do perineal anymore, we haven't done that for over 15 years, 100% are done robotic" I was relieved to hear that. So if you choose to research on youtube , then search for "robotic prostatectomy". That will most likely be what you will be getting.

Pre-Op Testing

Before surgery I had to do some pre-op testing. One was a pelvic MRI and the other was a full Bone Scan . Both were to determine if the cancer had spread outside of the prostate.

And the other 2 tests before surgery were a EKG to see if my heart can handle surgery and then 2 days before surgery I needed a COVID-19 test .

The MRI and Bone Scan were done at the hospital where the surgery would be done and the EKG was done at my primary care Dr office .

I thought the EKG was going to be like a heart "stress test" . Like hook me up with those little sticky sensors and run on a treadmill or ride an exercise bike for 20 minutes. No , not even close.
The nurse came in and put like 5 or 6 sticky sensors on me and turned on the EKG for maybe 15 seconds , and that was it… done.

The MRI and Bone Scan were different .
The MRI and Bone Scan were on 2 different days, I think they were 3 days apart . Not for any reason other than scheduling.

The MRI was focused on the pelvic area. So I did not have to be inside the MRI machine completely . I was only in the tunnel up to my chest area.
If any of you have done an MRI before , they are loud. I have done one many years ago for a shoulder injury.
The MRI technician gave me head phones and let me listen to whatever music I wanted to. The MRI was going to take 30 minutes.
I did have to undress into a gown, the imaging area gave me a locker to put my stuff in and they held the key for me in the MRI room.

When you go for your testing and appointments just take minimal belongings with you.

The Bone Scan was a little different. This was done in one day but required two visits to the hospital. The reason for this is I needed an injection of tiny radioactive tracers, then waited 3 hours and returned for the scan . You can learn more about bone scans <u>HERE</u> from the Mayo Clinic.

The technician doing the injection had some issues finding a good vein for the injection of the tracers. She went from my left arm to my right arm then finally to my left hand .

So with all that done and the covid test… I was ready for surgery on August 19th.

Some Emotions Start To Come Out

Before moving on I wanted to touch on something . Now in August 2020 this has been going on since my May 27th video visit about my high PSA Score. I haven't felt much emotion at all . I've been upset, kinda shocked, just going with , rolling with the punches.
I have contemplated my death , my mortality , not seeing my grandkids grow up and have kids.

The health care system we use has an app , and I use their app all the time. I can send my care team messages and they can message me . All my past and future appointments are on there and my test results and I can pay my co-pays there as well.

So after I did my MRI and Bone Scan , my test results came back on July 23rd . The formal test results written in medical field language , but my doctor added his own comment
" No evidence of cancer outside the prostate , Good News" my wife was napping in the bedroom, I walked in and told her , "It hasn't spread" and I just burst into tears . I couldn't stop crying . I layed down next to her and we both cried for a while.

I never cried like that before , and she never saw me cry like that . It was an unexpected emotional moment.

My Fears Of Surgery

My First Fear

I wanted to address this because it was relevant to me , and it may be relevant to you. I had never had surgery before. My biggest interaction with the medical community up to this point had been a broken foot and a shoulder injury.
I had never been under anesthesia at all, ever.

Everyone who had been under anesthesia is now giving me their story and for the most part it is regarding having their wisdom teeth pulled at the dentist. I guess my fear is going to sleep and not waking up . I find it unnerving being put out in one place and waking up in another and not being able to recall anything in between.

But the biggest fear about anesthesia was not waking up . Hey , it happens. People make mistakes. But of course this is going to happen , I had no choices at this point.

My Second Fear

My second fear I think may be every man's fear . It was having anything stuck up inside our penis. A catheter is my second fear . This was giving me major anxiety next to not waking up.
So what the surgeon and my urologist both told me was that it goes in while under anesthesia and comes out while you are awake.

So much of my thoughts were of the catheter removal day . I'll get into that later.

So those were my two fears that remained on my mind and gave me the most anxiety. Maybe yours as well , if so, you are not alone.

Surgery Day Is Here

August 19, 2020 , surgery day is here. My surgery was scheduled for 730am , I had to be there at 530am to get prepped by the surgical staff. Of course I wasn't the only one there. The hospital I was at does probably 60 to 70 surgeries per day .
So my wife drove me there in the morning and dropped me off. My fears of not waking up made it tougher saying goodbye to her. After we said goodbye I walked into the building. All I had with me was a small bag with my drivers licence , my insurance card , my cell phone and a pair of depends underwear.

The clothes I wore were just a t-shirt and pajama bottoms and my tennis shoes with no socks.

I walked into a lady checking temperatures in the lobby. Then I went to the surgery check in window. I checked in , signed 2 or 3 electronic forms and they sent me upstairs to my surgery waiting room.
I followed the instructions and headed upstairs . Nobody was around, I was the only one there. They must have known i was coming cuz just a few seconds after walking in the waiting room a lady came out and said , Ray ?
I said , yes.

She said come on in.

She was very friendly , and very comforting to me. Easy going was what I needed right then , and she was it.

She led me into a pre-op area , a wide hallway with open rooms down both sides. Each room had a hospital curtain . She took me to mine. I put my bag down on a chair and asked to use the bathroom.
She grabbed a new toothbrush and toothpaste and mouthwash and said , sure, follow me.

She said after you go to the bathroom, brush your teeth and use this mouthwash and spit it out.

When i was done I went back to my area and she came back in to give me some instructions.
She gave me a surgical gown , different from regular hospital gowns. She had some supplies with her . A couple of new blankets, surgical socks with rubber tread on them. She showed me everything and told me to undress and wash down my whole body with these giant , thick , warm wipes , and then put on the socks, the gown and relax.

I did that and layed down on the gurney and watched TV . There were 2 plastic bags, one for my clothes and belongings and one for my shoes.
I put my cell phone inside my tennis shoe. Then put the shoe bag inside the clothes bag .

All I can do now is wait.

I flipped through the channels on the TV and watched the local morning news. It was a Wednesday.
After a little while a nurse came in . Everyone who did anything with me first asked my name and birth date.
She came in to get the IV connection in and ready for the surgical team.

Then as the time got around 7am My Surgeon came in . He asked how I was doing and reassured me everything would be ok.

After he left a few minutes later my nemesis showed up . The anesthesiologist , he had a Australian or New Zealand accent , probably about the same age as me . I jokingly expressed my fears of not waking up. He understood and said it is very common to think that and he explained how it works.

He said once I'm all set on the operating table he would simply plug in the IV and deliver the anesthetic , most likely Propofol , but I didn't ask . He said he turns a dial one way and I fall asleep and then turns it back to wake me up. In between he just monitors my vital signs.

This will be a 4.5 hour surgery to remove my prostate, some surrounding lymph nodes and seminal vesicles.

After the anesthesiologist left the nurse came back in and told me , " I've been here for 20 years and he was here when I got here"

A short time later a man came in and pushed the curtain all the way open and he was there to take me to the operating room.
He made sure my stuff was following me , he put my stuff under the gurney, made sure no IV lines were hanging and he pulled my bed out of its room and started pushing me down the halls . We went into an elevator and went down , like to the basement down.

Down a hallway , the hallways were lined with gurneys and what I think was ventilators.
We stopped and he spun me around and backed us through a door into my operating room.

There was a young guy off to my left against the wall sitting at a desk . My surgeon was to my right looking at the DaVinci control center that he would be working at.

My anesthesiologist was there as well. The guy pushing me was in control at the moment and helped me move onto the operating table. Once I got comfortable on the operating table the anesthesiologist took over and asked If I was doing ok . I said yes.

And then I woke up .

4.5 hours had passed and I was upstairs in recovery and being cared for by nurses.

Very strange but I was glad it was over , compared to recovery the surgery was easy.

Overnight In The Hospital

Around 1pm I woke up in recovery, I honestly can't recall if I woke up while rolling to recovery or actually in my room.
I was in a double room , but I was by myself the whole time .
They had me on IV pain meds , I felt ok until I tried to move.

The goal overnight was for me to get up and walk 2 or 3 times. I ended up walking 2 times down the long hallway past the nurses station and back, I did that twice.
Once you're standing up it's ok , and once you're sitting down or laying down it's ok.

The hard part , the painful part is the transition from sitting to standing .

My condition was pretty good, I was not in any severe pain at all . On my own pain scale of 1 - 10 I was maybe a 3 . I know our own individual pain scales are different. Your 3 might be a 7 to me.
I can tell you this , stubbing my toe hurts way more than what I was feeling.

I had 6 incisions around my stomach . 5 small ones , maybe half inch each. And one a bit bigger , maybe 1 inch or so right above my belly button. That is the one they took the bad prostate out through. And the other bad tissue.
The incisions were not sewed or stapled , they were glued closed . So no return to have them removed. And at this point on August 30 , they are just fine. No leaking blood, no redness or any signs of infection. I am feeling much better today.

So there I was in recovery just resting. They brought me lunch. I was on a "clear" diet in recovery. It was a bowl of broth , chicken or beef. A pitcher of water, a cup of hot water and a tea bag. A cup of jello and another cup of jello like ice cream , it was great.
Same thing for dinner and breakfast the next morning.

Throughout the night the nurse came in with pain meds added to the IV and some I took with water, the techs came in to empty my catheter bag. When my phone died they charged it at the nurses station. I had a TV and an adjustable bed. I was pretty well cared for.
I did struggle to get up to a standing position to walk, but once I was up it was ok. I did take my walks as prescribed.

The overnight nurse was James , he was awesome from 6pm to 6am . He spent time with me and we talked. He was just a great nurse and really cared and was cool.

The next morning around 630am or so my surgeon showed up and went over how the surgery went with me. He said it went smooth as he expected. He was happy with everything. He told me he was happy with the removal of the prostate and surrounding lymph nodes and seminal vesicles.
He was also happy with the connection of the urethra to the bladder , which he tested in the operating room.

He gave me instructions for home again , to stay on clear liquids for the rest of the day . Then start eating whatever I want , just eat small bits and chew it up well before swallowing. Stay hydrated , drink a lot of water and good juices.
I was given Ibuprofen for pain 1 every 8 hours 600mg . I was also given Norco for pain as needed. (I didn't take any Narco at all)
I was given some for infection that I finished

And I was given a stool softener if I took Norco , because Narco can make you constipated.

My experience in this hospital was exceptional . They took such good care of me , very happy with the service.

They did not allow my wife up to visit me , but she was allowed to come up for catheter instruction right before we went home.

My wife showed up around 10am , and a veteran nurse just a few minutes later to talk to both of us about the catheter while at home. The catheter was going to be with me from the August 19th surgery day to August 25th .
Not too bad , pretty easy to take care of. Keep it clean around the entrance . Be mindful of any "tugging" on it . It works by gravity so make sure the bag and the path of urine is lower than your bladder.
I had 2 types of bags. The larger one that needed a place to put it while sitting on the couch or laying in bed.
And a smaller leg bag that needed more emptying , but made me mobile easier.

I switched to the leg bag for the ride home. The nurse gave us 3 leg bags and 2 extra big bags. She also gave us a bunch of hospital wipes to clean the entrance area, and sticky strips to hold the tubing to my thigh with slack so no tugging, designed for catheters.
A bunch of alcohol wipes for cleaning up the bag emptying tube.

After that 15 to 20 minute meeting we went home. The nurse came in and checked me out , a tech followed with a wheelchair .
The nurse gave me a pillow off the bed to take home and hold over my stomach for the ride.

TIP

The one thing I wish I took a couple of was the hospital gowns . 2 hospital gowns would have been awesome while dealing with the catheter for a few days. It would have made it much easier.
So grab 2 hospital gowns. Or at least stash the one you are wearing into your bag when you change clothes before you leave.

That was pretty much it. So Far , So Good … Right ?

First Day Back Home / My Catheter SetUp

When my wife and I got home I was still pretty medicated from the IV pain medication. One thing I did was make sure my wife picked me up at the hospital in my daughters Toyota Sienna minivan. I knew that would be much easier for me to get in and out of. Otherwise our cars are small cars much lower to the ground than the minivan.

So I pretty much got home and switched to the larger catheter bag and layed down in bed for a little while.
So after thinking and searching around for something to let the catheter bag hang on low to the ground without laying it on the ground, we came to this set up .

We took our bathroom trash can and lined it with a plastic trash bag . The large catheter bag has a plastic hook set up on it . It hung on the edge of the bathroom trash can perfectly. It just hung there inside the can lined with a clean new plastic trash bag. So when I get up I can just pick it up and take it with me to the restroom or the living room .

If I just want to walk around the house , the catheter bag also comes with a built in rope to hold it like a purse or bag. Instead of carrying the trash can .

You can see the plastic hook to hang and the rope to walk around at home.

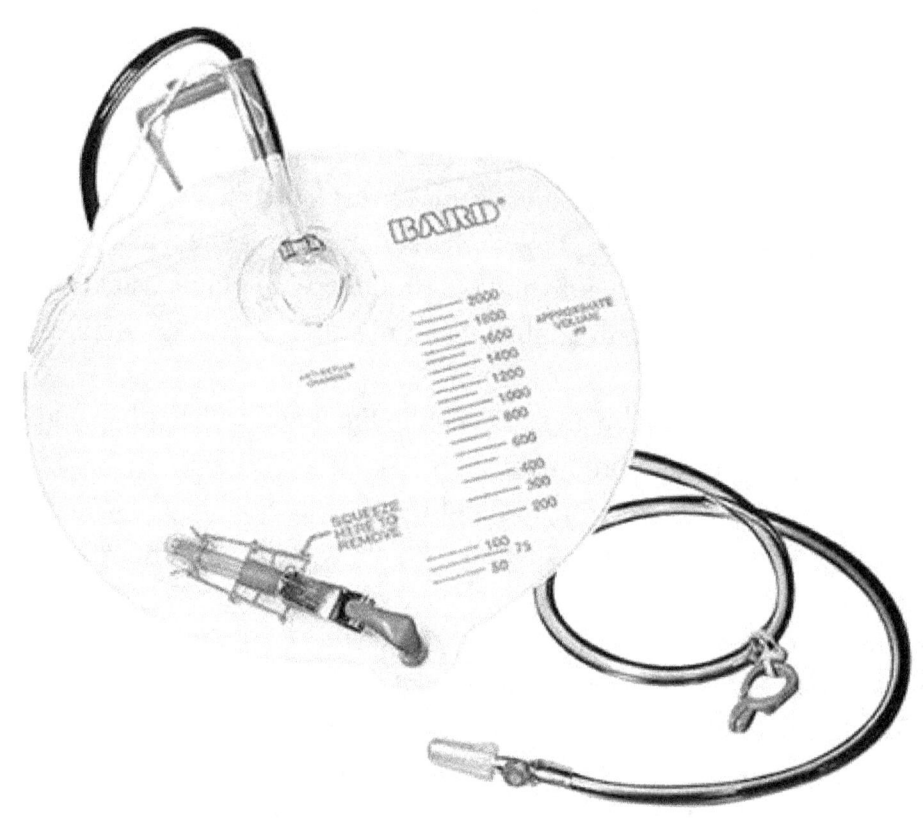

This is the exact catheter that I was given by my hospital . Most other catheters are very similar to this , with minor differences.

Here is the leg bag.

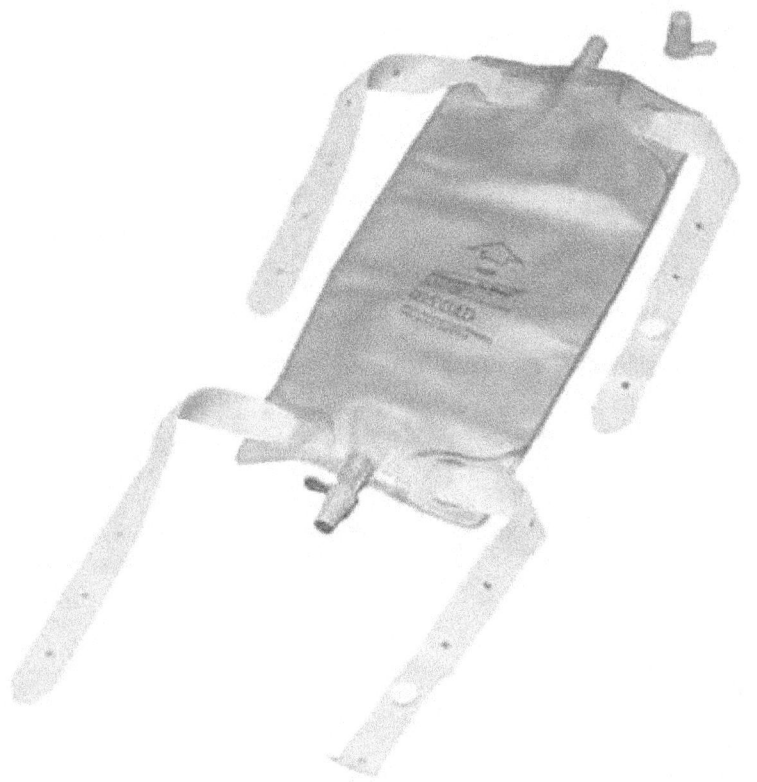

You just strap that to your thigh. When it fills up just undue the lower strap and aim the opening into the toilet. Then put the cap back on and redu the strap. Simple.

If you use a leg bag it is probably best with the hospital gown or really baggy basketball shorts, something like that, really loose fitting . Loose sweat pants would be good also.

The catheter wasn't as bad as I thought it would be, don't get me wrong , I didn't enjoy it . It was kind of convenient , hahaha .

So now it's August 19th around 3pm . I have until the 25th with the catheter. I will list all the things you should have at home ready for you at the end of this guide.

My first day home now. We got the catheter figured out for the house and I wish I had brought home a hospital gown right about now. Here's why. I want to use the larger bag so I don't have to empty as often. The big bag has the long tube so I need something loosely hanging like the gown . I had zero , nothing, so I wrapped a bath towel around myself when I was in our living room watching tv or something. I wrapped it and used a big chip clip or big file clip to hold it in place, so it wouldn't come undone and fall.

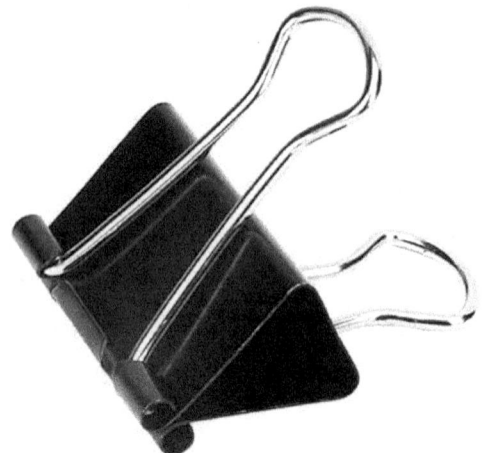

A clip like this to keep my bath towel on. If you forget the hospital gown and don't have really loose shorts. You'll understand why loose sweat pants don't work with the big catheter bag. A regular bathrobe would be just fine as well.

The care is pretty easy as well. The nurse who gave us the instruction said this.
Wash your hands often when dealing with your catheter.
After you drain the bag , use an alcohol wipe and wipe off the drain area before capping it or clipping it back in place.
That's pretty much it.

I was able to take showers since I had no stitches or staples. So I did. Showering with a catheter is no big deal , I just disconnected the bag and let the little rubber tube just dangle in the shower. It dripped a little urine while I showered , but that's ok.

When I was done I dried off and hooked back up the catheter and applied some Neosporin Plus Pain Relief to the entrance area , urethra . In case any unfortunate tugs . It keeps that entrance area lubricated and clean.

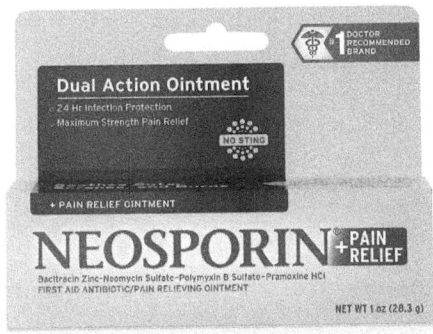

This being one of the items I will have on my list of must haves at home. That's pretty much it , now I'm ready for my 6 days at home with my new catheter !

Catheter Removal Day !

Alright ! , the last six days have been interesting to say the least . I was not in a lot of pain at all. So I did not take any of my Norco pain pills. And I stopped taking the ibuprofen as well .
I did have swelling around my penis and my testicles , but it has gone down .

The swelling around the shaft of my penis was on the right side and it was soft to the touch , it wasn't red or hard and did not hurt. I called the doctor about it and it was normal .

The testicle/scrotum swelling was normal as well.

As I write this guide it is August 30th and I'm 11 days now past my surgery on the 19th. The swelling is pretty much gone.

Okay so it is catheter removal day ! It was a 9am appointment on the 25th of August 2020.

So I put on a brand new leg bag and just wear pajama bottoms and a t-shirt to this appointment.

I arrived about 10 minutes early and they took me right in , maybe waited a few minutes.

A nurse assistant took my blood pressure and weight . She got the room ready for the nurse to do the removal.

The nurse came in and gave me a gown to wear and had me sit on the exam table. I was pretty nervous and ready for some kind of stinging pain to come on me. For some reason In my head I was imagining the same pain as when you get soap in your urethra when in the shower , only 10 times worse.

So she brings in some stuff , I notice a big sering like thing and a plastic bottle of clear solution and an empty container .

She has me lay back and she explains what she is going to do. She says ...

" I'm going to make sure you can pee on your own or the catheter will have to stay in" " so I'm going to fill your bladder with a clean saline solution and you're going to pee it out on your own" . I said OK.

So she removed the leg bag and the catheter just dangled out of my penis. She picked up the catheter and placed the big sering thing into the end of the catheter and filled the sering with the saline solution , and I watched it disappear into my bladder.

I can feel my bladder filling up. She said "When you feel like you have to pee , let me know"
I said OK , I have to pee .
She stood me up and held the empty container under my penis with the catheter dangling into the empty container.
I asked , are you going to pull out the catheter ? She said " No, your going to push it out with your pee"
And I looked down and started to pee normally and watched the catheter slide right out of my penis . Completely pain free .

I could not believe it. Everything I thought about a catheter was completely false. That was the best " Myth Busting" experience I ever had.

I thanked her and cleaned up . I bought a pair of mens large Depends with me in case I still leak a bit. I put them on and my pajama bottoms and waited for the doctor . My doctor who did the surgery came in and we went over some more things.

I told him and showed him the swelling and he did an exam and looked at the incisions and my penis and scrotum . He said everything looked good , the swelling will go down .
Asked me my experience with any pain . He basically told me this.
" Do a little bit more each day then the day before " and you will be fine.

Then he talked about the surgery. He told me he is still waiting on the pathology report for the lymph nodes and seminal vesicles he removed that were around and neatby the prostate.
We are hoping the cancer did not spread outside the prostate at all.

Now I mentioned earlier the MRI and Bone Scan pre operation showed no spread outside the prostate. But , microscopic cancer cells will not be visible to an MRI or bone scan.

It was a short visit, maybe 40 minutes total and it was good. The catheter is gone .

What I have noticed after the catheter removal is this. I do have a much better urine flow into the toilet. It does drip after I'm done peeing a bit more than usual.

And this is the issue I have that makes me wear Depends for a while longer. When I loosen up or push a little bit to pass gas … I leak , and it leaks quite a bit . So the Depends are also on my list of must haves. It does not have to be a Depends Brand… any adult protective garment is fine.

I might even switch to just a pad . We'll see how it goes and how the cost is different from a box of Depends to a box of pads. This is the one I got. Right now I am using one per day , changed out with a new pair every morning. I wear them just under my pajama pants . I have heard in some cases You can "leak" for a year. I hope not, we'll see.

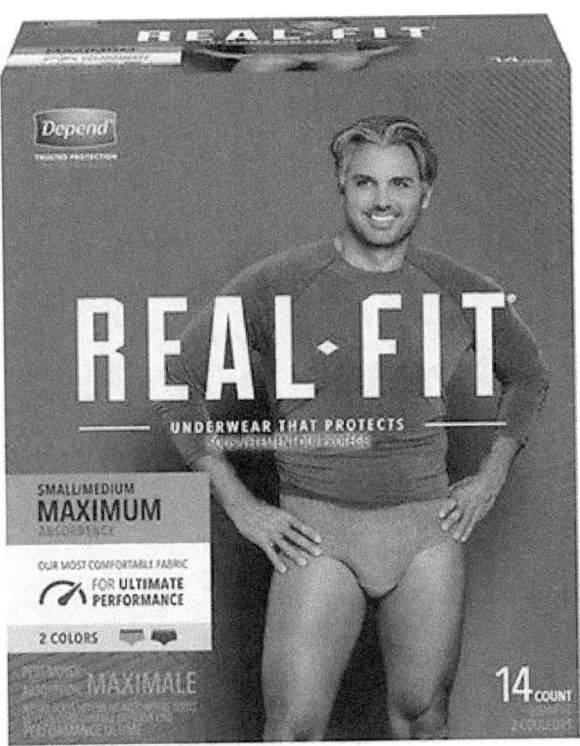

This is what I got .

Your Partner At Home

I must say that my partner at home has been my wife. We have been married for 15 years this month on August 27th. So much has been going on that we both missed it.
But I could not have done this well without her. Especially the first few days when it is nearly impossible to get up or lay down.

I needed her to hold on to me as I layed back into our bed , and help pull me up to a seated position. At least the first 2 or 3 days.
You really don't want to strain in those first few days.
She cooked for me and waited on all my needs.

I truly hope all of you have a helper / partner who can help you around those first few days , at least until you can sit and stand without straining.

I really have no idea what I would have done without her.

10 Days After Surgery

So here we are , 10 days after surgery . I'm actually feeling way better. I can do almost anything around the house. Now I am still careful , I can easily over do it and cause pretty severe pain. I really can't bend over and reach for things at certain angles. It still hurts .

I'm still not wearing jeans, I still just wear pajama pants all day long with depends underwear.

The incisions are scabbed over and at least 3 of them are right on my waste line where my jeans would be rubbing against and irritating the wounds.
I still brace for when I have to sneeze. At night if I have to sneeze I have a brace pillow I hold across my stomach . In fact that is the pillow I got from the hospital.

I have to say everything has gone really well , I am blessed with my wife and care team at the hospital.
The next step I am waiting for now is the pathology report of the tissue removed from around the prostate.

My Pathology Report Is Here

Anything removed from the human body within a medical setting is tested for disease. So all the tissue removed during prostate cancer surgery is tested and a pathology report is generated. This will tell you and your doctors if the cancer has spread outside of your prostate.

From what I was told from my first urologist was that almost 80% of men that have a prostatectomy due to prostate cancer will need additional treatment at some point , either sooner or later.

Well my pathology report was not good. The lymph nodes and seminal vesicles all tested positive for cancer. So this actually means the cancer has spread outside of the prostate.
So I will need additional treatment to "clean up" the area around the area around the prostate and where the prostate was.

I am going to do radiation treatment right after I heal up and get back to work.

Here is what I am told about any cancer . I'll use prostate cancer as an example. I can die of prostate cancer 15 years from now that spread to my lungs or bladder or brain or wherever. It is still prostate cancer.
If you are from New York and you move to California, you're still from New York .

So this is a pretty big blow to me, the fact that it spread outside the prostate brought tears to my eyes. I'm pretty upset. There is nothing I can do except move forward .

Helpful Supplies You Want At The House

1. Neosporin Plus Pain Relief
2. Depends or Equivalent
3. Chicken Broth
4. Beef Broth
5. Jello
6. Sorbet Ice Cream / Reg Ice Cream
7. Filtered Water
8. Pomegranate Juice
9. Berry Juice
10. Tea
11. Hospital Gown / Real Baggy Basketball Type Shorts
12. Bathroom / Office Type Plastic Trash Can
13. Plastic Trash Bag To Line Can
14. Wipes From Hospital
15. Alcohol Wipes From Hospital For Catheter ... Not Your Skin !
16. Flushable Wipes To Help Keep You Extra Clean Bowel Movement
17. Lip Balm From Hospital If Possible , Good Stuff
18. Pillow From Hospital For Sneeze Bracing.

Try to get everything and anything you can think of on this list and anything else you can think of. You don't need a lot of these things . Only for a week at most. You are going to feel way better after just 5 or 6 days.

Remember don't eat heavily the first couple of days home. Eat slow, chew real good. Stick with the clear foods day one and two. Broth, Jello, Juice, Water . Try one piece of toast to bind your stool.
We don't want you sitting on the bowl having huge bowel movements just yet.
Keep your penis and wounds clean . Wash your hands a lot and stay hydrated.

Wrap It Up , Where I'm At Today

I really hope this guide is a great value and helps you in the coming weeks for your prostate surgery. This has definitely been a learning experience .
My emotions and my wife's emotions have run the entire spectrum . It's been a real tough journey and we are just getting started.
I think this will be an ongoing issue for the rest of my life.

Where am I at right at this moment ? It's August 30th 745pm and I'm 11 days past my prostate cancer surgery.
I'm feeling way better each and every day. I'm still leaking when I feel I need to pass gas. And leaking a little bit after I think I'm done as I put everything back in my pants.

I've actually gained some weight since surgery. Maybe because I've been doing nothing. So I need to get busy and lose 15 pounds or so. I think the weight gain began back in mid July at the beginning of this cancer diagnosis.

I'd like to hear from all of you . Where are you at in your diagnosis? Has this guide helped at all ?
Do you just want to vent and talk about stuff ? Email me
prostatecancer1965@gmail.com

Here are some resources that can help you stay healthy and even someone young keep their prostate healthy.
All Natural Products , 3 of my favorites

http://www.lnk123.com/SH14k3
Curcumin anti inflammatory Inflammation is a killer

http://www.lnk123.com/SH14hi
Prostacet , healthy prostate for the next generation, give this to a young man in your life.

http://www.lnk123.com/SH14k4
Multi vitamin designed for men, if you are not taking a multivitamin, start now!

Thank you so much for downloading my Guide To Prostate Cancer

I hope it has helped you and God Bless You !

Ray
prostatecancer1965@gmail.com

Update !

So here I am , it's September 28, 2020 , about 40 days after surgery. I had a PSA test done on September 19 exactly 30 days after surgery.

What I'm told is that after a prostatectomy your PSA should be under .2 or basically undetectable. My PSA was .85 or over 4 times what it should be after surgery. It sucks.

So I had my appointment with my surgeon to discuss our treatment plan after getting this high PSA after surgery. At my appointment we talked about hormone therapy to lower my testosterone as much as possible since prostate cancer cells live on testosterone. And we talked about radiation.

I agreed on the hormone therapy and the radiation. Before I left his office I received a hormone injection. This injection was Eligard and it is a 3 month injection. So my next appointment to follow up on this is Dec 23rd. And I will get another PSA on Dec 19th. Hopefully it will be down dramatically.

As far as radiation goes I have referrals I need to call to meet with the oncologist. I will continue to update this.

2021

So here we are finally 2021 is here and we can maybe leave 2020 in the past. Many issues are going to linger with all of us for quite a while.

I hope you and your loved ones are doing ok.

I know the reason you purchased this book so I'm aware of the possible issues you or a loved one are facing.

So let me update this book with some info on where I am at right now. As I write this addition it is Feb 12, 2021 and I have been on hormone therapy (Zytiga) and Prednisone since Nov 18, 2020.

4 pills a day of the Zytiga and 1 Prednisone .

Then I began radiation treatment of my pelvic area to kill off any lingering cancer cells after surgery . The radiation treatments began on Jan 13, 2021 .

The way they do the radiation treatments is like this…

You go in every day Monday through Friday at a pre scheduled time for a short treatment. The entire treatment is only 5 minutes or even less.

You do this for 7 weeks , for me anyway.

As I write this I have completed 28 treatments. I have 11 left to go. Every Thursday for me I meet with my radiation oncologist to see how I am holding up during radiation.

So far It's been pretty easy and "event free" . Until Thursday Feb 4, 2020 .

That's when the nurses took my blood pressure and it rocketed up to 195 . They were worried about me having a stroke so they walked me over to the ER for some quick checks and tests not readily available in the radiation area.

I did an EKG and CAT Scan of my head. Nothing unusual so they gave me a blood pressure pill to lower my BP .
Medical Oncologist took me off that medication , the Zytiga and Prednisone and I have an appointment with him on the 17th of Feb.
I had a video visit with my primary care doctor to start me on blood pressure meds . I just picked that prescription up today and took the first pill.

So far elevated blood pressure has been my only serious side effect of hormone therapy. We definitely need to get that figured out because it is the hormone therapy that starves the cancer cells of testosterone.

As far as radiation goes I haven't really had any bad side effects at all. Let me tell you what the doctor told me just yesterday at my weekly meeting.

He said the first half of treatment is focused on just a small area , the area where my prostate used to be and a little bit around it.
The second half of the treatment goes to a much broader area , covering the bladder area and surrounding lymph nodes.
It is a low level radiation beam . It is the day after day of that low level beam that kills off cancer cells. The bad thing is it kills off all cells and causes inflammation and irritation.
The team of radiologists doing the treatment are great

people. I have complete confidence in them and I am not worried about them damaging my bladder or colon .

This afternoon , just about an hour ago I ate a M&M Ice cream sandwich . Bad Idea.
Diarrhea hit me hard for the first time since I began radiation. They warned me about it and told me to get some Imodium AD just in case.
They gave me a complete package about radiation treatment and what to expect and side effects . Even a nutrition plan of what to eat and what to avoid eating so I can reduce the chance of severe diarrhea .
Well now I know what they are trying to say.

My wife ran out to the store and bought me some Imodium AD . I got the liquid to drink . With just 2 weeks or so to go I need to be strict on my diet.
The doctor also told me that the second half is where most people start to feel some side effects of radiation. Treating a much bigger area will add to any possible effects of feeling bad.

So my 2 big concerns now is my blood pressure and the side effects of radiation treatment.

I truly hope you are getting some good info and value from my story. I will continue to add additions.